# HORMONE RESET DIET

## 40+ Breakfast, dessert and smoothie recipes designed for a healthy and balanced Hormone Reset diet

# TABLE OF CONTENTS

This document is geared towards providing exact and reliable information in regards to the topic and issue covered. The publication is sold with the idea that the publisher is not required to render accounting, officially permitted, or otherwise, qualified services. If advice is necessary, legal or professional, a practiced individual in the profession should be ordered.

- From a Declaration of Principles which was accepted and approved equally by a Committee of the American Bar Association and a Committee of Publishers and Associations.

## Introduction

Hormone reset recipes for personal enjoyment but also for family enjoyment. You will love them for sure for how easy it is to prepare them.

## BEANS OMELETTE

Serves:        **1**

Prep Time:    **5**    Minutes

Cook Time:   **10**   Minutes

Total Time:   **15**   Minutes

### INGREDIENTS

- 2 eggs
- ¼ tsp salt
- ¼ tsp black pepper
- 1 tablespoon olive oil
- ¼ cup cheese
- ¼ tsp basil
- 1 cup beans

### DIRECTIONS

1. In a bowl combine all ingredients together and mix well
2. In a skillet heat olive oil and pour the egg mixture
3. Cook for 1-2 minutes per side
4. When ready remove omelette from the skillet and serve

# ASIAN GREENS OMELETTE

Serves:          **1**

Prep Time:     **5**     Minutes

Cook Time:    **10**    Minutes

Total Time:    **15**    Minutes

## INGREDIENTS

- 2 eggs
- ¼ tsp salt
- ¼ tsp black pepper
- 1 tablespoon olive oil
- ¼ cup cheese
- ¼ tsp basil
- 1 cup Asian greens

## DIRECTIONS

1. In a bowl combine all ingredients together and mix well
2. In a skillet heat olive oil and pour the egg mixture
3. Cook for 1-2 minutes per side
4. When ready remove omelette from the skillet and serve

# BEANS OMELETTE

Serves:          *1*
Prep Time:    5    Minutes

Cook Time:    *10*    Minutes

Total Time:    *15*    Minutes

## INGREDIENTS

- 2 eggs
- ¼ tsp salt
- ¼ tsp black pepper
- 1 tablespoon olive oil
- ¼ cup cheese
- ¼ tsp basil
- 1 cup beans

## DIRECTIONS

1. In a bowl combine all ingredients together and mix well
2. In a skillet heat olive oil and pour the egg mixture
3. Cook for 1-2 minutes per side
4. When ready remove omelette from the skillet and serve

# CABBAGE OMELETTE

Serves:          *1*

Prep Time:     *5*    Minutes

Cook Time:    *10*   Minutes

Total Time:    *15*   Minutes

## INGREDIENTS

- 2 eggs
- ¼ tsp salt
- ¼ tsp black pepper
- 1 tablespoon olive oil
- ¼ cup cheese
- ¼ tsp basil
- 1 cup red onion
- 1 cup cabbage

## DIRECTIONS

1. In a bowl combine all ingredients together and mix well
2. In a skillet heat olive oil and pour the egg mixture
3. Cook for 1-2 minutes per side
4. When ready remove omelette from the skillet and serve

# MUSHROOM OMELETTE

Serves:        **1**

Prep Time:     **5**   Minutes

Cook Time:     **10**  Minutes

Total Time:    **15**  Minutes

## INGREDIENTS

- 2 eggs
- ¼ tsp salt
- ¼ tsp black pepper
- 1 tablespoon olive oil
- ¼ cup cheese
- ¼ tsp basil
- 1 cup mushrooms

## DIRECTIONS

1. In a bowl combine all ingredients together and mix well
2. In a skillet heat olive oil and pour the egg mixture
3. Cook for 1-2 minutes per side
4. When ready remove omelette from the skillet and serve

# TOMATO OMELETTE

Serves:      **1**

Prep Time:    **5**   Minutes

Cook Time:   **10**  Minutes

Total Time:   **15**  Minutes

## INGREDIENTS

- 2 eggs
- ¼ tsp salt
- ¼ tsp black pepper
- 1 tablespoon olive oil
- ¼ cup cheese
- ¼ tsp basil
- 1 cup tomatoes

## DIRECTIONS

1. In a bowl combine all ingredients together and mix well
2. In a skillet heat olive oil and pour the egg mixture
3. Cook for 1-2 minutes per side
4. When ready remove omelette from the skillet and serve

# OATS WITH PEANUT BUTTER

Serves:       **1**

Prep Time:    **5**   Minutes

Cook Time:   **5**   Minutes

Total Time:  **10**  Minutes

## INGREDIENTS

- 1 cup oats
- 3 tablespoons peanut butter
- ½ cup almond milk
- ¼ banana

## DIRECTIONS

1. In a bowl combine all ingredients together and mix well
2. Pour mixture into a jar
3. Refrigerate overnight
4. Serve in the morning

# BREAKFAST GRANOLA

Serves:        2

Prep Time:     5    Minutes

Cook Time:     30   Minutes

Total Time:    35   Minutes

## INGREDIENTS

- 1 tsp vanilla extract
- 1 tablespoon honey
- 1 lb. rolled oats
- 2 tablespoons sesame seeds
- ¼ lb. almonds
- ¼ lb. berries

## DIRECTIONS

1. Preheat the oven to 325 F
2. Spread the granola onto a baking sheet
3. Bake for 12-15 minutes, remove and mix everything
4. Bake for another 12-15 minutes or until slightly brown
5. When ready remove from the oven and serve

# BANANA PANCAKES

Serves:        **4**

Prep Time:   **10**   Minutes

Cook Time:   **20**   Minutes

Total Time:   **30**   Minutes

## INGREDIENTS

- 1 cup whole wheat flour
- ¼ tsp baking soda
- ¼ tsp baking powder
- 1 cup mashed banana
- 2 eggs
- 1 cup milk

## DIRECTIONS

1. In a bowl combine all ingredients together and mix well
2. In a skillet heat olive oil
3. Pour ¼ of the batter and cook each pancake for 1-2 minutes per side
4. When ready remove from heat and serve

# LIME PANCAKES

Serves:        *4*

Prep Time:    *10*  Minutes

Cook Time:   *20*  Minutes

Total Time:   *30*  Minutes

## INGREDIENTS

- 1 cup whole wheat flour
- ¼ tsp baking soda
- ¼ tsp baking powder
- 1 cup lime
- 2 eggs
- 1 cup milk

## DIRECTIONS

1. In a bowl combine all ingredients together and mix well
2. In a skillet heat olive oil
3. Pour ¼ of the batter and cook each pancake for 1-2 minutes per side
4. When ready remove from heat and serve

# GUAVA PANCAKES

Serves:        *4*

Prep Time:    *10*   Minutes

Cook Time:    *30*   Minutes

Total Time:   *40*   Minutes

## INGREDIENTS

- 1 cup whole wheat flour
- ¼ tsp baking soda
- ¼ tsp baking powder
- 2 eggs
- 1 cup milk
- 1 cup guava

## DIRECTIONS

1. In a bowl combine all ingredients together and mix well
2. In a skillet heat olive oil
3. Pour ¼ of the batter and cook each pancake for 1-2 minutes per side
4. When ready remove from heat and serve

# APRICOT MUFFINS

Serves:        *8-12*

Prep Time:     *10*    Minutes

Cook Time:     *20*    Minutes

Total Time:    *30*    Minutes

## INGREDIENTS

- 2 eggs
- 1 tablespoon olive oil
- 1 cup milk
- 2 cups whole wheat flour
- 1 tsp baking soda
- ¼ tsp baking soda
- 1 tsp ginger
- 1 cup apricot
- ¼ cup molasses

## DIRECTIONS

1. In a bowl combine all dry ingredients
2. In another bowl combine all dry ingredients
3. Combine wet and dry ingredients together
4. Pour mixture into 8-12 prepared muffin cups, fill 2/3 of the cups
5. Bake for 18-20 minutes at 375 F

6. When ready remove from the oven and serve

# PEACH MUFFINS

Serves:        **8-12**

Prep Time:     **10**    Minutes

Cook Time:     **20**    Minutes

Total Time:    **30**    Minutes

## INGREDIENTS

- 2 eggs
- 1 tablespoon olive oil
- 1 cup milk
- 2 cups whole wheat flour
- 1 tsp baking soda
- ¼ tsp baking soda
- 1 tsp cinnamon
- 1 cup mashed peaches

## DIRECTIONS

1. In a bowl combine all dry ingredients
2. In another bowl combine all dry ingredients
3. Combine wet and dry ingredients together
4. Pour mixture into 8-12 prepared muffin cups, fill 2/3 of the cups
5. Bake for 18-20 minutes at 375 F
6. When ready remove from the oven and serve

# BLUEBERRY MUFFINS

Serves:        *8-12*

Prep Time:    *10*   Minutes

Cook Time:   *20*   Minutes

Total Time:   *30*   Minutes

## INGREDIENTS

- 2 eggs
- 1 tablespoon olive oil
- 1 cup milk
- 2 cups whole wheat flour
- 1 tsp baking soda
- ¼ tsp baking soda
- 1 tsp cinnamon
- 1 cup blueberries

## DIRECTIONS

1. In a bowl combine all dry ingredients
2. In another bowl combine all dry ingredients
3. Combine wet and dry ingredients together
4. Fold in blueberries and mix well
5. Pour mixture into 8-12 prepared muffin cups, fill 2/3 of the cups
6. Bake for 18-20 minutes at 375 F

7. When ready remove from the oven and serve

# PAPAYA MUFFINS

Serves:      *8-12*

Prep Time:   *10*   Minutes

Cook Time:   *20*   Minutes

Total Time:  *30*   Minutes

## INGREDIENTS

- 2 eggs
- 1 tablespoon olive oil
- 1 cup milk
- 2 cups whole wheat flour
- 1 tsp baking soda
- ¼ tsp baking soda
- 1 tsp cinnamon
- 1 cup papaya

## DIRECTIONS

1. In a bowl combine all dry ingredients
2. In another bowl combine all dry ingredients
3. Combine wet and dry ingredients together
4. Pour mixture into 8-12 prepared muffin cups, fill 2/3 of the cups
5. Bake for 18-20 minutes at 375 F
6. When ready remove from the oven and serve

# CORN OMELETTE

Serves:         *1*
Prep Time:    *5*    Minutes

Cook Time:   *10*   Minutes

Total Time:   *15*   Minutes

## INGREDIENTS

- 2 eggs
- ¼ tsp salt
- ¼ tsp black pepper
- 1 tablespoon olive oil
- ¼ cup cheese
- ¼ tsp basil
- 1 cup corn

## DIRECTIONS

1. In a bowl combine all ingredients together and mix well
2. In a skillet heat olive oil and pour the egg mixture
3. Cook for 1-2 minutes per side
4. When ready remove omelette from the skillet and serve

Serves:          *1*

Prep Time:    *5*    Minutes

Cook Time:    *10*    Minutes

Total Time:    *15*    Minutes

## INGREDIENTS

- 2 eggs
- ¼ tsp salt
- ¼ tsp black pepper
- 1 tablespoon olive oil
- ¼ cup cheese
- ¼ tsp basil
- 1 cup mushrooms

## DIRECTIONS

1. In a bowl combine all ingredients together and mix well
2. In a skillet heat olive oil and pour the egg mixture
3. Cook for 1-2 minutes per side
4. When ready remove omelette from the skillet and serve

# YAMS OMELETTE

Serves:        *1*

Prep Time:    *5*    Minutes

Cook Time:   *10*   Minutes

Total Time:   *15*   Minutes

## INGREDIENTS

- 2 eggs
- ¼ tsp salt
- ¼ tsp black pepper
- 1 tablespoon olive oil
- ¼ cup cheese
- ¼ tsp basil
- 1 cup yams

## DIRECTIONS

1. In a bowl combine all ingredients together and mix well
2. In a skillet heat olive oil and pour the egg mixture
3. Cook for 1-2 minutes per side
4. When ready remove omelette from the skillet and serve

# RAISIN BREAKFAST MIX

Serves:        **1**

Prep Time:     **5**     Minutes

Cook Time:     **5**     Minutes

Total Time:    **10**    Minutes

## INGREDIENTS

- ½ cup dried raisins
- ½ cup dried pecans
- ¼ cup almonds
- 1 cup coconut milk
- 1 tsp cinnamon

## DIRECTIONS

1. In a bowl combine all ingredients together
2. Serve with milk

# SAUSAGE BREAKFAST SANDWICH

Serves:       2

Prep Time:    5    Minutes

Cook Time:   15   Minutes

Total Time:  20   Minutes

## INGREDIENTS

- ¼ cup egg substitute
- 1 muffin
- 1 turkey sausage patty
- 1 tablespoon cheddar cheese

## DIRECTIONS

1. In a skillet pour egg and cook on low heat
2. Place turkey sausage patty in a pan and cook for 4-5 minutes per side
3. On a toasted muffin place the cooked egg, top with a sausage patty and cheddar cheese
4. Serve when ready

# STRAWBERRY MUFFINS

Serves:        *8-12*

Prep Time:    *10*   Minutes

Cook Time:    *20*   Minutes

Total Time:   *30*   Minutes

## INGREDIENTS

- 2 eggs
- 1 tablespoon olive oil
- 1 cup milk
- 2 cups whole wheat flour
- 1 tsp baking soda
- ¼ tsp baking soda
- 1 tsp cinnamon
- 1 cup strawberries

## DIRECTIONS

1. In a bowl combine all dry ingredients
2. In another bowl combine all dry ingredients
3. Combine wet and dry ingredients together
4. Pour mixture into 8-12 prepared muffin cups, fill 2/3 of the cups
5. Bake for 18-20 minutes at 375 F
6. When ready remove from the oven and serve

# LEEK FRITATTA

Serves:       *2*

Prep Time:    *10*   Minutes

Cook Time:    *20*   Minutes

Total Time:   *30*   Minutes

## INGREDIENTS

- ½ lb. leek
- 1 tablespoon olive oil
- ½ red onion
- ¼ tsp salt
- 2 ggs
- 2 oz. cheddar cheese
- 1 garlic clove
- ¼ tsp dill

## DIRECTIONS

1. In a bowl whisk eggs with salt and cheese
2. In a frying pan heat olive oil and pour egg mixture
3. Add remaining ingredients and mix well
4. Serve when ready

# KALE FRITATTA

Serves:      **2**

Prep Time:   **10**  Minutes

Cook Time:  **20**  Minutes

Total Time:  **30**  Minutes

## INGREDIENTS

- 1 cup kale
- 1 tablespoon olive oil
- ½ red onion
- ¼ tsp salt
- 2 eggs
- 2 oz. cheddar cheese
- 1 garlic clove
- ¼ tsp dill

## DIRECTIONS

1. In a skillet sauté kale until tender
2. In a bowl whisk eggs with salt and cheese
3. In a frying pan heat olive oil and pour egg mixture
4. Add remaining ingredients and mix well
5. Serve when ready

# GREENS FRITATTA

Serves:        *2*

Prep Time:    *10*   Minutes

Cook Time:   *20*   Minutes

Total Time:   *30*   Minutes

## INGREDIENTS

- ½ lb. greens
- 1 tablespoon olive oil
- ½ red onion
- ¼ tsp salt
- 2 eggs
- 2 oz. parmesan cheese
- 1 garlic clove
- ¼ tsp dill

## DIRECTIONS

1. In a bowl whisk eggs with salt and parmesan cheese
2. In a frying pan heat olive oil and pour egg mixture
3. Add remaining ingredients and mix well
4. Serve when ready

# BROCCOLI FRITATTA

Serves:        **2**

Prep Time:   **10**   Minutes

Cook Time:   **20**   Minutes

Total Time:   **30**   Minutes

## INGREDIENTS

- 1 cup broccoli
- 1 tablespoon olive oil
- ½ red onion
- ¼ tsp salt
- 2 oz. cheddar cheese
- 1 garlic clove
- ¼ tsp dill

## DIRECTIONS

1. In a skillet sauté broccoli until tender
2. In a bowl whisk eggs with salt and cheese
3. In a frying pan heat olive oil and pour egg mixture
4. Add remaining ingredients and mix well
5. When ready serve with sautéed broccoli

# _DESSERTS_

## BREAKFAST COOKIES

Serves:          **_8-12_**

Prep Time:     **5**     Minutes

Cook Time:     **15**    Minutes

Total Time:     **20**    Minutes

### INGREDIENTS

- 1 cup rolled oats
- ¼ cup applesauce
- ½ tsp vanilla extract
- 3 tablespoons chocolate chips
- 2 tablespoons dried fruits
- 1 tsp cinnamon

### DIRECTIONS

1. Preheat the oven to 325 F
2. In a bowl combine all ingredients together and mix well

3. Scoop cookies using an ice cream scoop
4. Place cookies onto a prepared baking sheet
5. Place in the oven for 12-15 minutes or until the cookies are done
6. When ready remove from the oven and serve

# BLUEBERRY PIE

Serves:        *8-12*

Prep Time:     *15*   Minutes

Cook Time:     *35*   Minutes

Total Time:    *50*   Minutes

## INGREDIENTS

- pastry sheets
- ¼ tsp lavender
- 1 cup brown sugar
- 4-5 cups blueberries
- 1 tablespoon lemon juice
- 1 cup almonds
- 2 tablespoons butter

## DIRECTIONS

1. Line a pie plate or pie form with pastry and cover the edges of the plate depending on your preference
2. In a bowl combine all pie ingredients together and mix well
3. Pour the mixture over the pastry
4. Bake at 400-425 F for 25-30 minutes or until golden brown
5. When ready remove from the oven and let it rest for 15 minutes

# PUMPKIN PIE

Serves:      *8-12*

Prep Time:   *15*   Minutes

Cook Time:   *35*   Minutes

Total Time:  *50*   Minutes

## INGREDIENTS

- pastry sheets
- 1 cup buttermilk
- 1 can pumpkin
- 1 cup sugar
- 1 tsp cinnamon
- 1 tsp vanilla extract
- 2 eggs

## DIRECTIONS

1. Line a pie plate or pie form with pastry and cover the edges of the plate depending on your preference
2. In a bowl combine all pie ingredients together and mix well
3. Pour the mixture over the pastry
4. Bake at 400-425 F for 25-30 minutes or until golden brown
5. When ready remove from the oven and let it rest for 15 minutes

# RICOTTA ICE-CREAM

Serves:        *6-8*

Prep Time:    *15*   Minutes

Cook Time:   *15*   Minutes

Total Time:   *30*   Minutes

## INGREDIENTS

- 1 cup almonds
- 1-pint vanilla ice cream
- 2 cups ricotta cheese
- 1 cup honey

## DIRECTIONS

1. In a saucepan whisk together all ingredients
2. Mix until bubbly
3. Strain into a bowl and cool
4. Whisk in favorite fruits and mix well
5. Cover and refrigerate for 2-3 hours
6. Pour mixture in the ice-cream maker and follow manufacturer instructions
7. Serve when ready

# SAFFRON ICE-CREAM

Serves:        *6-8*

Prep Time:    *15*    Minutes

Cook Time:    *15*    Minutes

Total Time:    *30*    Minutes

### INGREDIENTS

- 4 egg yolks
- 1 cup heavy cream
- 1 cup milk
- ½ cup brown sugar
- 1 tsp saffron
- 1 tsp vanilla extract

### DIRECTIONS

1. In a saucepan whisk together all ingredients
2. Mix until bubbly
3. Strain into a bowl and cool
4. Whisk in favorite fruits and mix well
5. Cover and refrigerate for 2-3 hours
6. Pour mixture in the ice-cream maker and follow manufacturer instructions
7. Serve when ready

# *SMOOTHIES*

## TURMERIC-MANGO SMOOTHIE

Serves:          **1**

Prep Time:    5    Minutes

Cook Time:    5    Minutes

Total Time:    **10**    Minutes

### INGREDIENTS

- 1 cup Greek yogurt
- ¼ cup orange juice
- 1 banana
- 1 tablespoon turmeric
- 1 tsp vanilla extract
- 1 cup ice

### DIRECTIONS

1. In a blender place all ingredients and blend until smooth
2. Pour smoothie in a glass and serve

# AVOCADO-KALE SMOOTHIE

Serves: **1**

Prep Time: **5** Minutes

Cook Time: **5** Minutes

Total Time: **10** Minutes

## INGREDIENTS

- 1 cup coconut milk
- 1 tablespoon lemon juice
- 1 bunch kale
- 1 cup spinach
- ¼ avocado
- 1 cup ice

## DIRECTIONS

1. In a blender place all ingredients and blend until smooth
2. Pour smoothie in a glass and serve

# BUTTERMILK SMOOTHIE

Serves:        **1**

Prep Time:     **5**   Minutes

Cook Time:     **5**   Minutes

Total Time:   **10**  Minutes

## INGREDIENTS

- 1 cup ice
- 1 cup strawberries
- 1 cup blueberries
- 1 cup buttermilk
- ½ tsp vanilla extract

## DIRECTIONS

1. In a blender place all ingredients and blend until smooth
2. Pour smoothie in a glass and serve

Serves: *1*

Prep Time: 5 Minutes

Cook Time: 5 Minutes

Total Time: *10* Minutes

## INGREDIENTS

- 1 cup berries
- 1 cup baby spinach
- 1 tablespoon orange juice
- ¼ cup coconut water
- ½ cup Greek yogurt

## DIRECTIONS

1. In a blender place all ingredients and blend until smooth
2. Pour smoothie in a glass and serve

# FRUIT SMOOTHIE

Serves:      **1**

Prep Time:   5   Minutes

Cook Time:   5   Minutes

Total Time:  **10**   Minutes

## INGREDIENTS

- 1 mango
- 1 cup vanilla yogurt
- 2 tablespoons honey
- 1 tablespoon lime juice
- 1 banana
- 1 can strawberries
- 1 kiwi

## DIRECTIONS

1. In a blender place all ingredients and blend until smooth
2. Pour smoothie in a glass and serve

Serves: **1**

Prep Time: **5** Minutes

Cook Time: **5** Minutes

Total Time: **10** Minutes

## INGREDIENTS

- 2 cups mango
- 1 cup buttermilk
- 1 tsp vanilla extract
- 1 cup kiwi
- ½ cup coconut milk

## DIRECTIONS

1. In a blender place all ingredients and blend until smooth
2. Pour smoothie in a glass and serve

# DREAMSICLE SMOOTHIE

Serves:      **1**

Prep Time:    **5**   Minutes

Cook Time:    **5**   Minutes

Total Time:   **10**   Minutes

## INGREDIENTS

- 1 cup Greek yogurt
- 1 cup ice
- ¼ cup mango
- 1 orange
- 1 pinch cinnamon

## DIRECTIONS

1. In a blender place all ingredients and blend until smooth
2. Pour smoothie in a glass and serve

# FIG SMOOTHIE

Serves:         **1**

Prep Time:    **5**    Minutes

Cook Time:   **5**    Minutes

Total Time:   **10**   Minutes

## INGREDIENTS

- 1 cup ice
- 1 cup vanilla yogurt
- 1 cup coconut milk
- 1 tsp honey
- 4 figs

## DIRECTIONS

1. In a blender place all ingredients and blend until smooth
2. Pour smoothie in a glass and serve

# POMEGRANATE SMOOTHIE

Serves:        **1**

Prep Time:    **5**   Minutes

Cook Time:   **5**   Minutes

Total Time:   **10**   Minutes

## INGREDIENTS

- 2 cups blueberries
- 1 cup pomegranate
- 1 tablespoon honey
- 1 cup Greek yogurt

## DIRECTIONS

1. In a blender place all ingredients and blend until smooth
2. Pour smoothie in a glass and serve

# GINGER-KALE SMOOTHIE

Serves:        **1**

Prep Time:     **5**    Minutes

Cook Time:     **5**    Minutes

Total Time:    **10**   Minutes

## INGREDIENTS

- 1 cup kale
- 1 banana
- 1 cup almond milk
- 1 cup vanilla yogurt
- 1 tsp chia seeds
- ¼ tsp ginger

## DIRECTIONS

1. In a blender place all ingredients and blend until smooth
2. Pour smoothie in a glass and serve

**THANK YOU FOR READING THIS BOOK!**

CPSIA information can be obtained
at www.ICGtesting.com
Printed in the USA
BVHW031703160321
602551BV00027B/305